Richard Adams is a retired primary school headteacher, artist, author, broadcaster and playwright. Born in Northamptonshire, his career took him to Norfolk and Lancashire, and his retirement took him to Leicestershire and Lancashire for a second time. His wife's dementia brought him to Nottingham to be closer to family. They have a son, a daughter, and four grandchildren.

For Chris, even though she won't know why, and for all those who care for loved ones with dementia.

Richard Adams

ARE YOU MY HUSBAND?

Thirty Conversations with Dementia

AUSTIN MACAULEY PUBLISHERS™

LONDON • CAMBRIDGE • NEW YORK • SHARJAH

A CIP catalogue record for this title is available from the British Library.

ISBN 9781035843329 (Paperback)
ISBN 9781035843336 (ePub e-book)

www.austinmacauley.com

First Published 2024
Austin Macauley Publishers Ltd®
1 Canada Square
Canary Wharf
London
E14 5AA

Table of Contents

Author's Note   9

1: Small Talk   10

2: Does a Pig Know It's a Pig?   12

3: Dreams and Disinclination   14

4: Mirror, Mirror   16

5: Fair Shares   18

6: Keeping in Touch   20

7: Keep Taking the Tablets   22

8: Driven to Distraction   24

9: Pillow Talk   26

10: Needs No Ironing   28

11: The Trouble with Pork Pie Salad   30

12: Evening Out   32

13: Safety and Security   34

14: Sleepyhead   36

15: To Have and To Hold   38

16: At Work   40

17: Bath Lift   42

18: Thighs   44

19: Independence   46

20: Work to Be Done   48

21: Shopping   50

22: All by Myself   52

23: Out of Sorts   54

24: Tulips   56

25: Money for the Loo   58

26: Out for Lunch   60

27: Sorry, Sorry, Sorry   62

28: Nobody Knows – Part One   64

29: Nobody Knows – Part Two   66

30: Trees in the Corners   68

Author's Note

In 2019, my wife developed a combination of Alzheimer's and vascular dementia. For four years, I have been her full-time carer. I have retained my sanity by getting up early and writing for a couple of hours. It is a kind of therapy before I go into the bedroom and announce that I am thinking of getting breakfast. My wife has lost the will and the ability to attend to the usual household chores. Sometimes she does not remember who I am.

I have slowly come to understand that no one case of dementia is alike and that there is no one-size-fits-all way of dealing with it. This is my own personal – sometimes very personal – approach.

These thirty conversations and reflections record episodes in our relationship and how dementia has impacted upon our lives. I have treated them, I hope, with honesty and sensitivity but also with humour, not to make light of what is a difficult experience but to encourage anyone who is in a similar situation to enjoy a moment of recognition, to smile, even to laugh, but above all, to find encouragement to keep going and be undefeated by the mysterious illness called dementia.

Richard Adams

May 2023

1
Small Talk

There is a shortage of conversation in our household. Since there are only the two of us, there is hardly likely to be a constant hubbub, and since my wife and I have been married for sixty years, it's hardly surprising that topics of conversation are somewhat limited; added to which, we moved house in the middle of the pandemic, which prevented us from making contacts, so we can't even gossip about the neighbours.

But the main reason for the absence of conversation is that my wife has dementia. Things we might have conversations about rely on memory, and memories elude her.

"Are you my husband?"

"Yes," I say.

"Mmm," she says, "I thought you might be."

But sometimes she '*does*' know. If she goes to the loo but forgets what to do when she gets there, she will call for me. "Richard, can you help me?" So, I will go to find her and give her instructions.

"You are good to me," she says, as though I were a live-in carer, not her husband and lifelong companion.

"How long have we been married?"

"Sixty years."

"Have we really? You poor thing."

"Why am I a poor thing?" I ask.

"Having to look after me. I'm sorry to be such a burden."

"You're not a burden," I tell her. "It's what husbands are for. You know, in sickness and in health, for richer or for poorer, for better or for worse, till death us do part."

"Not all husbands," she says, and I marvel at that moment of lucid perception.

Sometimes there are windows in the otherwise blank wall of her memory. It gives me a shiver of delight when one of them opens, and the sunlight that once glowed in the girl I fell in love with over sixty years ago, suddenly brightens the day of a husband who has unexpectedly become her full-time carer.

2

Does a Pig Know It's a Pig?

"When we go home," my wife says, "we must take that with us. It's mine."

"What is?" I ask.

She points to a papier mâché pig, which she made at an adult craft class many years ago. It sits on the floor in front of the TV and appears to be looking quizzically at the two of us as we sit together on the sofa.

"Oh," I say, "the pig."

"It's not a pig," she says. "It's a dog."

It has piggy ears, a piggy snout and is bright pink. "I thought it was a pig," I say, "but you made it, so if you say it's a dog, it must be a dog."

"It's a dog," she insists. "I'll take it home."

The received wisdom is that you don't contradict a person who has dementia on the grounds that it will increase their confusion. I don't always heed the advice. In fact, I sometimes challenge it.

"Where will you take it if you take it home?" I ask.

"To my parents' house," she replies.

Rather than bluntly tell her that her parents are long dead, I try to get her to work it out for herself.

"How old are you?" I ask.

"I don't know."

"Date of birth?" I ask, knowing that there is an automatic response to this resulting from regular visits to the Warfarin Clinic.

"Twenty-five, twelve, thirty-five," she says, but she can't do the maths, so I tell her she is eighty-seven and point out the unlikelihood of her parents still being alive.

"Besides," I add, "you can't take the pig home. It's already home. This is where we live. This is home. This is our house. You live here. I live here. We are at home. The pig is at home."

"It's a dog," my wife says.

Sometimes you can't argue with the certainty of dementia, but tomorrow, or even in ten minutes, the dog might be the pig it really is.

3

Dreams and Disinclination

"Have you got any money?"

I force my eyes open and emerge from a deep sleep.

"What?"

"Have you got any money?"

My wife is bending over me, one hand on the bed to stop herself from toppling over. It is nearly three o'clock in the morning. "What do you want money for?"

"To pay for the things at the door."

"What things?"

"I can't remember, but I have to pay for them."

"I think you must have been dreaming. Get back into bed. We'll sort it out in the morning."

When I get up about eight and go downstairs, every light is on, every door wide open. A packet of rice is out of the kitchen drawer and sits on the worktop. Other food packets have been rearranged. A blood pressure monitor, still in its box, has been transferred to a small table in the lounge. Whatever she was dreaming of has been re-enacted downstairs. I return all the items to their rightful places.

About ten, I return to the bedroom and suggest that it's time for breakfast.

"Are you bringing it up here to me?" my wife asks.

For a long time, I have resisted this. It is difficult to know if her reluctance to get out of bed is genuine physical pain and frailty due to arthritis and a heart condition or what I have come to label D.D.D.: Dementia-Driven Disinclination.

"You can't stay in bed forever," I tell her. "I don't want you to become a permanently bedbound old woman, withering away until you die. I want you to have a day that's been worth living, even if it's only coming down for breakfast. You were up half the night, up and downstairs, trying to pay for goods at the door you'd only dreamt about. You're not an invalid."

"You're cross with me," she says.

The truth is, I'm cross with myself for losing my rag because dementia doesn't care, so I needn't have wasted my breath.

4

Mirror, Mirror

"Stir your stumps," I tell my wife.

"Why?" she says. "What's happening?"

"You have a hair appointment."

"Where?"

"At the hairdressers."

"Where is it?"

"It's in the middle of a row of shops on Dungannon Road, but you're no nearer now, are you?"

"No," she answers. "I can't picture it."

Dementia has deprived her of what was once a vivid photographic memory.

"What do I have to do?" she asks, and I have to spell out each step of the way.

"Get up, get washed, get dressed, have some lunch, and then I will push you to the hairdresser's in the wheelchair."

It takes an age, with some assistance, for her to carry out these instructions, but at last we have finished our coffee and sandwiches and are ready to go.

At the hair salon, Collette is pleasant and attentive, but as I look at my wife's reflection in the mirror as Collette cuts, combs and tweaks stray hairs into place on the head of an eighty-seven-year-old, I am tempted to ask why I make the effort to get her there. If the weather is not wheelchair-friendly, a taxi there and back almost doubles the price of a hairdo.

But I know why. Some women let themselves go. If dementia ruled, my wife would be let go, unkempt and dishevelled. The first thing she asks for when I have helped her get dressed is a comb.

At the salon, she looks in the mirror, and I see her smile. Then Collette swings her around in the chair, and my wife says, "Will I do?"

"You'll do splendidly," I say.

There is an elegant piece of signwriting on the salon wall that reads, "Be your own kind of beautiful."

Dementia may have robbed my wife of a great many things, but self-esteem is not going to be one of them.

5

Fair Shares

Lying next to me in bed, my wife is making strange murmuring sounds. Suddenly, she pulls herself up and sits on the edge of the bed.

"What are you doing?" I ask her.

"I've got something in my stomach," she says. "Do you want it?"

I translate the reference to the contents of her stomach as meaning she has a full bladder.

"Do you need the loo?" I ask her.

"I think so," she says, "but I've got all this liquid. I thought you might want some." Dementia has made her generous to a fault.

"Thank you, but no," I say. "I've plenty of my own. Go to the loo and flush it down the pan." She does as she's told, and when she gets back, I no longer face the prospect of an unsolicited gift.

"You, OK?"

"Yes, I think so," she says, and gets back into bed.

Dementia seems to have a way of unearthing things from childhood. I suspect that my wife, like most children, was encouraged to share – sweets, toys, games – but not I hope the contents of her bladder. Dementia mixes things inappropriately.

At mealtimes, I give her less than a child's portion of the main course because she has an appetite problem. "That may well be cognitive," the doctor had said.

By the time I have cleared my plate, my wife is still picking and choosing from the food on hers. "Would you like some of this?" she asks, pushing her plate towards me.

"I'd sooner you ate it," I say. "You've only had one Weetabix and half a banana. You'll fade away from lack of sustenance."

"I can't eat any more," she says.

I sometimes think it's less to do with appetite than botheration. I take away the plates and serve the dessert. Strangely, there appears to be no appetite problem when the food on offer is vanilla cheesecake. She won't share that with anybody.

6

Keeping in Touch

"Are we sleeping here tonight?" my wife asks.

"Yes," I say.

She asks, "Is there a bed?"

"Yes."

"Where?"

"In our bedroom," I tell her, deliberately including 'our' because I know what's coming next.

"What do you mean, *our* bedroom?"

"We've been sleeping together for over sixty years," I say.

"Do my parents know about it?" she asks.

I don't imagine her parents gave our sleeping together much thought other than the prospect of becoming grandparents, but since that was sixty years ago and now that they are dead, they are unlikely to think about it at all, but my wife's dementia does not distinguish between then and now.

"Where is it?" she asks. She means the bedroom.

"Up the stairs, first door on the left. Where we slept last night...and the night before that, and the night before that...and the night before that..."

I have got used to repeating myself. Every night, after the TV six o'clock news – sometimes in the middle of it – she asks where we're sleeping. She cannot grasp that twenty months ago we moved house and have been sleeping in our new home ever since. She expects to 'go home' to sleep somewhere else. Every night, I contradict this notion.

Other notions that require answers repeatedly are about the children.

"Have you put the children to bed?"

"No."

"Are you going to meet the children out of school?"

"No."

The 'children' are fifty-seven and fifty-eight, with children of their own.

I retain my sanity by trying to frame my answers in as many different ways as possible. It is at least a way of communicating. I have a friend who visits someone with dementia in a residential care home and only asks her if she knows how lovely it is in Abu Dhabi, Abu Dhabi, Abu Dhabi, over and over.

With my wife, despite the misunderstandings and confusion, there is at least a two-way conversation. I rejoice that we are still connecting.

7

Keep Taking the Tablets

"What are these for?" my wife asks, looking at two tablets in the palm of her left hand.

I have just put them there, and a small glass of water in her right hand with which to wash them down.

I point at them. "That one is to reduce cholesterol, and that one to reduce your blood pressure."

"Why?"

"They will help to prevent you from having a heart attack or a stroke," I tell her.

"How do you know that?"

"I've read the leaflets in the pill boxes."

"Who says I have to take them?"

"The doctor."

Long before the onset of her dementia, my wife was diagnosed with atrial fibrillation. She takes five pills a day, which are intended in one way or another to thin her blood and keep her heart beating rhythmically. A sixth pill is to stop the nerve endings in her brain from becoming even more tangled than they are.

One night, after an episode of *Miss Marple*, in which the murder victim had been poisoned with thallium, my wife took exception to her bedtime pills.

"I'm not taking those," she said. "You might be trying to poison me."

I couldn't persuade her otherwise, so the pills went unswallowed. Next day, we were back to normal, but by teatime, she was questioning again, "What are these for?"

"One for your blood, one for your brain," I tell her.

The prescription record says 'Indefinitely'. I order them online and dispense them day in day out, only now and again stopping to wonder what would happen if I didn't do it anymore, if I were to give up the medication routine that is serving to keep her alive, inhabiting a confused and purposeless life. I don't know whether or not it would precipitate her death. I do know I'm too afraid to risk it, and even with all the demands on my time and energy, or even because of them, I would miss her terribly.

8

Driven to Distraction

"Can we go and visit one of the family?" my wife asked.

She had seen the sun shining. Our daughter lives but a half-hour's drive away. It's an opportunity to get my wife dressed and out for a while. For me, it is an opportunity not to be missed. Looking after a wife with dementia can be inhibiting. I need to get out too.

But…and it was big but.

"We can't just get up and go," I said. "We don't have a car anymore."

"Why not?"

"We no longer have a car. I sold it."

"Why?"

"Neither of us can drive anymore," I said. "The DVLA have revoked my licence. My eyesight is no longer good enough."

"*I* can drive," she said.

"No, you can't," I said.

"I can," she insisted.

The DVLA have not been told that my wife has dementia. Her licence has simply lapsed, but I didn't let her drive. She can't always find her way about the house, let alone be trusted with a car on the highway. Anyway, I've sold it.

She used to drive competently to Flower Club, W.I. and church meetings. If I had been more alert, I might have suspected the beginnings of dementia long before the final diagnosis. She was late home one night.

"Where have you been?" I said.

"I got lost," she said.

"How can you have got lost?" I asked. She'd made the same journey innumerable times.

"I must have taken a wrong turn," she said. "Then I found myself by Morrison's roundabout, and I remembered where to go."

It's only now I see how that was probably the first signs. If only, with the benefit of hindsight, we could turn back time and put a stop to what becomes unchangeable.

"I'm glad you're safe," I said.

9
Pillow Talk

"Where are we?" my wife asks.

"In bed," I reply.

"Yes," she says, "but where?"

"In our bedroom."

"Yes," she says again, "but where?"

"At home."

"Where's home?"

I recite our full home address, even including the postcode, but she is not done yet.

"Are we in England?"

I'm tempted to add what I used to write in a new book when I was a child, where there was a space inside the front cover headed 'This book belongs to…' where I would complete the address with 'England, United Kingdom, Europe, the World, the Universe, Outer Space'. My wife's dementia-driven question does not seem to have a satisfactory answer.

"Do we live here?"

"Yes."

"Are we married?"

"Yes."

"That's a relief."

"Why?" I want to know. It's not the first time we have lain in bed and she has asked these questions. My theory is that she thinks we are living in a guest house. We could be anywhere, but as long as she is in bed with her husband, it must be OK. She will come down to breakfast and ask, "Just the two of us?"

"Yes, just you and me."

"Where are the others?"

"There are no others," I reply. "We are at home. You live here. I live here. Just you and me. Nobody else."

"Are you my husband?" she says.

"Yes, I say."

"Mmm, I thought you'd say that."

It is not only that dementia has robbed her of her memory. It has also robbed her of self-confidence. She requires repeated reassurance. She cannot be sure that she knows what she thinks she knows. I repeat what I've told her almost every day since her dementia afflicted her so quickly that the doctors were amazed at the speed of her deterioration. I remind her of the date of our wedding, the name of the church and the town in which it took place.

"I'm not sure that's true," she says, and I silently scream.

10

Needs No Ironing

"I think you'd better have a bath," I tell my wife.

"Am I smelly?" she asks.

"Just a bit," I tell her, which is putting it mildly. I can't believe she hasn't noticed. Spasmodic incontinence doesn't help, but she has acquired an infection that makes matters worse.

At eighty-seven and despite an arthritic hip, she is surprisingly capable of getting in and out of the bath, so I leave her in bed and go to run it and tell her when it's ready. I make sure she lowers herself into the water without skidding over and leave her to it. Sometimes she will appear at the bathroom door, dried and towel-wrapped, shiny clean and smelling sweet, but on this occasion, she calls for help. Her brain seems to have lost the ability to tell her body what to do. I suspect it's a combination of the infection and dementia, but she can't manoeuvre so as to pull herself up by the grab rail and stand up. I try to assist her, but she is too heavy, and a slithery wrestling match ensues. If we were fifty years younger, it would be fun, but in the end, we dialled 111 for advice, and they called for paramedics who managed the task between them. We have now installed a bath lift.

Through all of this, I am reminded of the old joke in which an old woman streaks naked across a football pitch. One spectator says, "Who's that?"

His mate says, "No idea, but she needs ironing."

I have always admired my wife's back. It is smooth and beautiful, and even in the midst of the tussle and tears of getting her out of the bath, it was a joy to behold, and I was moved to reflect that even in adversity, there are miracles. At eighty-seven, it still needs no ironing.

11

The Trouble with Pork Pie Salad

"It's time we had some lunch," I tell my wife.

She is still in bed, where earlier I had given in to her refusal to get up and served her breakfast at about 10.30 a.m.

"It's nearly two o'clock," I say.

No response, so I persist, "I'm getting pork pie salad."

She pulls herself up, looks at me and says, "It's too heavy."

"What do you mean it's too heavy?" She has no answer.

"I'll go and get it," I say. "Will you come downstairs?"

I'm not very hopeful. Yesterday, I had the same problem. I had explained that the cleaners were due and would want to clean the bedroom and that a neighbour was calling in for a cup of tea about three o'clock, an event that I hoped would brighten her day and persuade her that it was worth getting up.

I prepare the salad, my wife's portion: two thin slivers of pork pie, a small heap of shredded lettuce and two small tomatoes. The kitchen table with its red cloth and shining tumblers looks as though it belongs in a classy bistro. I do try. I envisage the two of us sharing a pleasant lunch.

As I go upstairs, I catch her already out of bed, but she is only on her way to the loo. When she emerges, I offer her a bathrobe and invite her to come down.

"That's too heavy," she says and slides back into bed, sitting up as though expecting a meal.

"You're expecting me to bring it up, then. Why?"

"Why not? It's warm and cosy here."

"It's warm and cosy in the kitchen," I say. "The sun is shining."

"Perhaps I don't want any lunch."

"Not ever again?" I ask her.

She doesn't reply. Defeated, I bring lunch upstairs.

An expert once said you should never speak of people 'suffering' from dementia. Call it an illness. Fine, but the person with dementia doesn't know she has dementia. Whereas the carer knows and feels it all too well.

.

12

Evening Out

"What day is it?" my wife wants to know.

"Wednesday," I tell her.

"What's happening today?" she says.

I list the day's agenda. "Breakfast, then I'm going for a haircut. Snack lunch, a bath for you, then you get dressed, ready to go out."

"Where to?"

"We're going out for a meal, then to the theatre."

I repeat this throughout the day to keep her on track and persuade her to comply with all the demands of getting ready for an evening out. "Liz is coming with us," I say.

"Who's Liz?"

"Our daughter."

"Do I know her?" she asks.

"You should," I say. "You gave birth to her."

"Really?"

"Yes, really. Fifty-eight years ago. When she was eighteen, she left home for college and hasn't been back since, except to visit, and we've been to visit her. It's because of her that we moved to live where we do now so that she's on hand if I find myself struggling to look after you. She's only half an hour away by car. When we lived in Blackpool, it was three hours up the M6."

"I can't picture her."

"I know."

"Is she married?"

"Yes; we have grandchildren."

"Do we really?"

Our daughter arrives, but it does nothing to restore my wife's memory. "You look familiar," she says, "but I can't quite place you."

Despite this, the evening out is a good one: a fine meal and a stunning performance by Theatre de Complicite. My wife and I sit, holding hands. She is mostly silent, and I don't know whether she is engrossed or simply failing to engage. Sometimes watching TV at home, it is evidently not capturing her mind, but tonight is different. When we get home, she says, "That was a good event." She may not recognise our daughter, but now and again, she knows a good time when she has one. I rejoice that all is not completely lost.

13
Safety and Security

"What are you looking for?" my wife asks.

"My phone," I say. "I'm sure I had it here."

My wife is sitting up in bed, having just had breakfast on a tray. I had mine from a tray at the foot of the bed. I have now cleared the breakfast things away and taken them downstairs into the kitchen, but in the process, my smartphone has gone missing.

"What does it look like?" my wife asks.

"It's black, like a thin wallet," I say.

"Is that it?" she asks, pointing to the TV remote.

"No," I say, "that's for the television."

I go downstairs and look in every ground-floor room. It's not there. I traipse back upstairs and look in my small office, even in the bathroom, but it's not there either. The only solution is to ring myself up using the landline phone, so I do and hear my smartphone ringing in the bedroom.

I finally track it down to the pocket of my wife's bathrobe, which she had put on while I was dealing with the breakfast things.

"What's it doing there?" I ask. "You must have 'tidied it up' for me," I say.

"I didn't put it there," she says.

I stop myself from saying, 'You must have done' because I know she simply doesn't remember doing it. It wouldn't be the first time. We spent ages looking for her electric toothbrush and only found it days later in a little-used handbag. Her dementia seems to have evoked an enhanced sense of security. Gadgets apparently just lying about need to be moved to a place of safety.

She seems obsessed with drawing the curtains in the lounge, not to deter prying eyes but to stop the light from the room from escaping into the street. I detect a moment of throwback to the 'blackout' requirements of the war. Dementia appears to have no sense of chronology.

14
Sleepyhead

"What are we doing?" my wife asks.

"Sitting on the sofa," I say.

"No. What are we doing?" she says again. Her dementia doesn't always allow her to say exactly what she means. I translate it as wanting to know what we're going to do for the rest of the evening.

"We could play Scrabble," I suggest.

"What's Scrabble?"

We played Scrabble for sixty years, but she has lost interest in anything requiring mental focus, and now it appears she has forgotten what Scrabble is.

"I expect we'll watch the telly," I say.

"Is there anything on?"

Inwardly, I despair at the multiplicity of choices. "I expect we can find something, and at some point, I'll get a little supper."

"That'll be nice," she says, "and then we can go to bed."

"Well, eventually, yes. It's only half past six."

"I'm so tired," my wife says.

Boredom may have something to do with it. I wonder if, like her lack of appetite, her tiredness is cognitive. We watch an old episode of *Vera*, but she seems disengaged.

"What time is it?" she asks.

"Quarter past eight. I'll get some drinks and nibbles," which I do while the adverts are on.

"What a feast," my wife says. "Are the others coming to have some?"

I have put together some oddments from the fridge: sausage rolls, chunks of cheese, pieces of apple and fruit juice.

"There is no one else," I tell her. "Just you and me."

She only picks at the food. "I want to go to bed," she says.

"Then you'd better go," I say. "But I'm going to see the end of this programme." I see her up the stairs and into bed. "I'll see you about ten," I say.

When *Vera* has ended, I clear away the supper things and take my wife's bedtime medication up to her. She is not asleep. She has not slept at all, but bed is somewhere to be warm and cosy and to pass the time with no demands that challenge her dementia's disinclinations.

15

To Have and To Hold

I have nodded off in an armchair. When I open my eyes, my wife is staring at me.

"I'm trying to work out who you are," she says.

"Have you come to any conclusion?" I ask.

There is a long silence, and I wonder which of the several possible answers she will offer me because it's not the first time she has wondered who I am. Answers have included her son, her father, her cousin and 'some bloke who lives here'. Her dementia will not allow her to find the words for 'full-time' live-in carer.

At last, she says, "I was hoping you'd tell me."

"I'm your husband, Richard."

"You don't look like Richard."

"So, you keep telling me, but I am."

"Are we married?"

"Yes," I say, and repeat, for the umpteenth time, the day, the date and the place of our wedding. I take her hand and point to the wedding ring. "I gave you that," I tell her.

"Do we have any children?"

"We have two. One's fifty-eight and the other's fifty-seven."

Somewhere in her dementia-infected mind, I can tell the cogs are whirring, and a surprising possibility clicks into place.

"Do we sleep together?"

"Every night for the last sixty years," I say, "and if we've got two children, then we must have had sex at least twice."

"Ooh," she says, feigning embarrassment and putting her hands over her face. Then, after a pause, she peeps at me through her fingers and giggles. It is one of those rare moments when I realise dementia has not entirely deprived her of her sense of humour, and, best of all, she knows who I am and who it is she is able to share such moments with.

16
At Work

My wife is on the move. She has switched on the bedside lamp and is standing at the end of the bed.

"What are you doing?" I ask.

"I'm looking for the materials," she says.

"What materials?"

"They're sort of shiny," she says.

"Like baking foil?"

"No," she says, and returns to sit on the edge of the bed, opening and shutting the drawers of the bedside chest, searching for the materials.

"I think you've been dreaming," I say. "And now you've woken up. What you saw in your dream isn't there anymore."

She is not to be convinced. "You're the one who's dreaming," she says. "We can't do the work without the materials."

"Come back to bed, and let's get some sleep," I say.

"I didn't come here to sleep. I came to work. I suppose you're just going to lie there sleeping, and we'll get nothing done!"

When her frustration has subsided, she gets back into bed. We sleep for an hour or so when I hear her say, "Nothing gets done that way."

I don't query it. When you are your wife's full-time carer, sleep is too precious. She dozes off again anyway.

I don't get back to sleep. I lie awake wondering where such dreams come from – dreams that move my wife to act out the circumstances of them. I try to think of past events that may have suddenly resurfaced, but if that's what they are, they may well have been events that took place before we met.

In any case, as a writer, I know that the brain is a repository of original thought. Past history isn't necessarily essential to generate a new story. In spite of, or because of, my wife's dementia, she has a source of creativity that, if I could but harness and understand it, could well be the beginnings of a new play or a novel. That mysterious creativity may be as much in me as it is in her and has nothing at all to do with dementia.

17
Bath Lift

"Ooh," my wife says. "That's posh."

We are standing in the doorway of the bathroom, and she is commenting on the bath lift. It is not new. She has used it several times before, but dementia deprives her of the memory.

"I've run the bath," I say. "Better get in it before it gets cold."

"What do I have to do?" she asks.

"Better take your nightie off first," I suggest.

"Oh, and my watch."

"Yes," I say. "I'll put it in my pocket."

She pulls her nightie over her head and begins to clamber over the edge of the bath.

"No," I say. "Hang on. See if the water's OK; not too hot."

She paddles her hand in the water and says it's OK. Then she tries once more to climb in.

"Not like that," I say. "You'll topple in," and I repeat the instructions for the bath lift.

"Turn around and sit on that flap." She does so. "Swing your legs over the side."

"Like this?"

"Yes. Spot on. Now, ease yourself into the middle of the seat."

When she is in position, I press the button on the handset, and the lift slowly and gently descends.

"This is fun," she says, as though she's never done it before.

So, I join in. "Going down," I say, "Haberdashery, Menswear, TV and Electricals," as though descending in the lift of an old-fashioned department store.

We laugh together, and she is finally in the water, warm, relaxed and lying back contentedly as though the memory loss and confusion of her dementia were a million miles away.

"This is lovely," she says. "What a shame I have to get out."

"Take as long as you like," I say, running in some more hot water. "We don't have a bus to catch."

"That's as well," she says, looking at her naked body.

And we laugh some more.

18
Thighs

"How are you this morning?" I ask my wife.

"My leg hurts," she says.

If her dementia were not enough to contend with, she is also troubled with arthritis.

"Is it a cocodamol day?" I ask.

"What's cocoda…coco…whatever you said?"

"It's a painkiller," I say, "or I could rub some ibuprofen gel on it."

"Whatever." She shrugs.

The cocodamol tablets are downstairs, so I opt for the Ibuprofen gel lying in its fat tube on the chest of drawers. My wife hitches up the hem of her nightdress to reveal her smooth thigh. For an eighty-seven-year-old, it is surprisingly shapely, firm and smooth.

"You could play Principal Boy in Panto, you know?"

"What are *you* after?" she says with a mischievous grin, dementia momentarily subdued to reconnect us.

"If only," I say to myself. "Where do you want this gel?"

She eases her nightdress further up and runs her hand along her thigh. "Just here," she says, and after a pause, "I think."

I squeeze a line of gel along her thigh and begin to rub it in. "Is that the right place?" I ask.

"I don't know. I think so. It's bloomin' cold."

"It's meant to be," I say. "To numb the pain. Does it still hurt?"

"I don't know."

No. She doesn't know, and neither do I. When I mentioned my wife's lack of appetite to the doctor, he said it could be 'cognitive'. It makes me wonder if the pain in her thigh might also be 'cognitive'. It comes and goes, but it's *her* leg, so who am I to know if it hurts or not? When she prefers breakfast in bed to coming downstairs for it, sympathy competes with suspicion. More often than not, it's sympathy that wins.

19

Independence

"Do I put sugar on this?" my wife says.

She has in front of her a single Weetabix in warm milk. A bowl of sugar is beside it.

"Yes," I say. "I like to grant you a degree of independence."

I suddenly regret saying that. It's sarcastic and unnecessary. My wife's dementia often removes the ability to make decisions, even to carry out simple functions like sugaring her Weetabix or preparing vegetables. Sometimes I invite her into the kitchen when I'm getting lunch.

"How would you like me to cut these carrots?"

"You decide," I say. "Slice them lengthways into batons, diagonally into lozenges or chop them into discs. You choose."

"No," she says. "Tell me how you want them doing."

"Like this," I say, and demonstrate. She follows suit. Uninstructed, she would continue to flounder.

Sometimes, if she seems up to it, I will suggest we go out for lunch.

She can dress herself but asks, "What shall I wear?"

"Bra, top, trousers, shoes," I say, taking them out of the wardrobe and laying them on the bed.

In the restaurant, the waiter asks, "Drinks?"

My wife looks at me. "What shall I have?" Once she would have ordered lemonade, but she drinks very little, and almost a glassful would be returned to the kitchen and poured down the sink. I resent the cost of this, so I order tap water.

"Shall we share a starter?" I ask. No reply.

"So much choice," she says. "I don't know where to start."

"Whitebait?" I suggest. One portion, two forks. The waiter is accommodating. We have been before, and he knows that my wife has an appetite problem, which obliges us to share a single three-course meal.

Choosing for herself is something she has lost the confidence to do. I shouldn't mock. Fortunately, she won't remember that I've been sarcastic. I would love for her to be less dependent on me, but dementia has decreed that's not how it is.

20

Work to Be Done

"Am I depriving you of any of these things?" my wife says.

"What things?" I ask, sitting up in bed. She is sitting on the edge of the bed and has cleared all the bits and bobs from her bedside chest of drawers.

"What are you doing?"

"Getting ready for work," she says.

"It's five o'clock in the morning," I tell her.

When she leaves the bedroom, I assume she is going to the loo, but she takes a long time to return, so I get up and find her in the guest room, about to get into bed.

"Please don't," I say. "If you sleep there, I shall have to strip the bed and wash the bedclothes."

"I need the space," she says, sweeping a hand across the duvet, "for the work."

"Not at five o'clock in the morning," I say, and steer her back to bed.

She arranges her pillows so that she can sit up. Then she begins to explain.

"We need to sort those clothes," she says.

She is able to dress herself, but when she undresses before bed, she simply dumps her clothes on a bedroom chair. There is a great heap that I haven't had the will or the energy to sort and hang back in the wardrobe. The 'work' she refers to is to lay the clothes on the bed and sort them into those that need re-hanging and those that need to go in the wash. She can do this better in the guest room since there will be no lump of a husband in the bed.

"I don't want to disturb you," she says.

For a woman with dementia, it is a surprisingly logical and lucid explanation, but I can do without it at five in the morning.

"OK," I say, "but it's too early. We need to sleep. Let's attend to it in the morning."

"All right," she says reluctantly, and settles down.

In the morning, the heap of clothes is still there, and the 'work' that was so urgent entirely forgotten.

21
Shopping

"I'm going to do the shopping," I tell my wife.

"Where?" she says, rubbing her eyes.

It is 7.30 a.m. If I get up early and leave her in bed, I can do the weekly shop and know that she is safe.

"Look at you," she says.

It's a cold morning, and I've put on my thick red anorak.

"Turn around," she says, so I do a twirl.

"This is my shopping expedition outfit," I say, and she laughs, her dementia lifting for a moment to let her enjoy the daftness that married couples sometimes share. Despite the early hour, she is surprisingly bright. *Will it last?* I wonder.

"I'll be about an hour," I tell her.

"Have a nice time," she says.

When I return, I park the groceries in the kitchen and go upstairs to tell her I'm back. I meet her as she comes out of the bedroom.

"There's nobody about," she says. "I was just going downstairs. Is there any breakfast?"

"Well, it's early," I say, "but we can have breakfast now if you like."

Usually, she stays in bed until about ten while I do some household chores or work in my office.

At breakfast, she asks, "Where are the others? Have they gone to work?"

"There's just you and me," I tell her. "This old married couple. No one else lives here."

At lunchtime, she eats surprisingly well. Sausage and mash. "Would you like me to pay for this?" she asks.

"When we got married," I explain, "we opened a joint account. My pension and yours go into it. It pays for the council tax, the gas, the electricity, the shopping and anything else we need."

She looks unsure. After lunch, we move into the lounge. I sit with my back to the window, my face in shadow.

"Are you my husband?" she says.

Such a bright start, but steadily downhill from then on. "Frailty," I mutter, "thy name is dementia."

I move to sit beside her, and she puts her hand in mine.

22

All by Myself

"Is there anybody there?" my wife calls up the stairs. I'm tempted to ask if she's conducting a séance.

"I'll be down shortly," I reply. "I need to finish an email."

"You're always in that office," she says. "Don't be long."

Her dementia forgets that I need to escape into my office to write, to lose myself in the dialogue of a playscript or email a friend, but mostly to be 'me'.

I go downstairs. She is sitting in the lounge.

"It's good to have your company," she says.

I have only been gone for twenty minutes. "Was there something you wanted?" I ask.

"I was lonely," she says.

"Shall I put the telly on?"

"I don't want the noise," she says.

"Cup o' tea?"

"That would be nice."

So, I make some tea, and we sit together on the sofa.

"Are you my husband?" she says.

"Yes."

"I thought you'd say that. I don't see you very often."

"We were in bed together, all night," I say.

"We can't see each other in bed," she says with an undemented flash of humour.

I try again. "We had breakfast together; we had a coffee mid-morning; we had lunch together. I accept you were on your own while I got the lunch. I can't be with you all the time, or nothing would get done."

"I could do things," she says, "but you don't let me."

"You're ill," I say. "You can't do the things you used to do. I've been doing them for the last four years."

"Have you really?" she says. "That must be hard. You are good to me."

"I know," I say, but when she complains that she is lonely, I sometimes wish I could be lonely too. Just for a while.

23

Out of Sorts

"How are you this morning?" I ask my wife.

She is curled up foetus-like in the bedclothes. She squints at me. "I don't know how I feel. Peculiar. I'm not normal."

I refrain from being facetious. "Where are you not normal? Head? Leg? Stomach?"

"I can't display," she says. "No, that's not right, is it?"

"I think *explain* is the word you're looking for," I say. "Ache? Pain? Feeling sick? Perhaps you need something to eat. I'll get the breakfast."

"All right," she says, and begins to wrestle herself out of the duvet.

As she sits on the edge of the bed, I see that she's right. Something is not normal. She went to bed in a nightdress. She is now in a bathrobe and naked under it.

"I haven't got any knickers on," she says.

No, she hasn't, and there's no sign of them anywhere. I find her nightdress on the floor. It is wet.

"Have you wet the bed?" I ask. She checks the sheet. It's dry. In any case, the nightdress doesn't smell of pee. Most nights, her wanderings wake me up. For once, I must have slept right through. I've no idea what she's been doing in the middle of the night.

"What have you been doing? How did your nightdress get wet?"

"I don't know," she says.

At least she has managed the situation somehow without my assistance; she removed her nightdress, put on a bathrobe and got herself back into bed. In the dark!

It's a mystery.

I find her some clean pants and nightdress. I put the wet nightdress to be washed and ignore the mystery. "Stay positive," I tell myself. "Dwelling on the negative will lead to despair, and you'll become a bitter old man, resentful and full of self-pity. No. Stay positive. It's the only way to stay sane. Possibly the only way to treat dementia."

24
Tulips

"Who sent those flowers?" my wife asks, pointing to a pot of beautifully handcrafted tulips above the fireplace. I decide to challenge her dementia and see if she can work it out for herself.

"They were a Mother's Day gift," I say. "So, who might have sent them?"

"Did you send them?"

"You're not my mother," I say. "You're eighty-seven, and I'm eighty-two. Is it likely?"

"Oh, *I know*," she says, so pleased that she has remembered because she knows that she forgets things, and then she falters, "No, it's gone."

"Who are you a mother to?" I ask.

"Erm...two," she says.

"That'll do for a start," I say. "Which one sent the tulips?"

"My cousin," she says. Dementia is like a library where the books keep falling off the shelves.

"No," I say. "You have a son called Jon. He sent them." Then I correct myself. "*We* have a son called Jon."

I should have left well alone. The conversation now goes in a different direction.

"We?" she says. "Are we married?"

"Yes."

"To each other?"

"Yes."

"I don't think that's true."

"I know you don't," I reply. "But it *is* true, whether you think it is or not. It's your illness that makes you think otherwise."

"You're making things up," she says.

"No," I say. "You make things up because it's what dementia makes you do."

"What's dementia?" she asks.

"It's an illness," I say. "It makes your brain dysfunctional. You imagine things. You forget things. You get confused."

"Will I get better?" she wants to know.

I hesitate before I answer because I'm not sure I want to give her a blunt 'No'. The consolation is that we have been talking to each other, maintaining a loving and respectful relationship, and in a short while, she'll have no memory of what I say. So, I say it, "No. You take pills to stop it from getting any worse, but no, no cure."

"I suppose that's better than nothing," she says.

25

Money for the Loo

I am just nodding off nicely in an armchair after lunch when my wife says, "I haven't got any money."

"What do you need money for?" I ask.

I haven't told the bank that my wife has dementia and doesn't know any longer how to manage money. They still renew her debit card. It comes in handy for spreading Polyfilla.

"If I'm going to the toilet," my wife says, "won't I need some money?"

Her mind is confusing the downstairs toilet with a public convenience requiring coins in a slot to gain entrance. How does dementia do that? And why? Dots get joined up that shouldn't be joined up.

Often, wherever she goes, she wants to take her handbag. Before dementia (B.D.), it was an essential accessory. It still is, except it has no money in it. It may have a lipstick and a comb, but only if she's remembered to put them back after she's used them. It once had an electric toothbrush in it. We'd been looking for it everywhere and had bought a new one before we found it. Anything she didn't know what to do with would be given a home in the handbag until it was bursting at the seams. It was only a small black clutch bag, but it was bulging like an overstuffed pillow, hanging by a leather loop from her wrist and clumping against her walking stick, threatening to cause a fall.

"Will I need my handbag?" she says as we prepare for an outing.

"No," I say. "I've got money and a comb and lipstick in my pocket if you need them."

I don't tell her that in a bag that hangs on the back of the wheelchair, I have spare incontinence pants, a towel and a supply of plastic bags.

Dementia with diplomacy.

26
Out for Lunch

"Are we having any lunch today?" my wife asks. She has noticed it is 12.30. It is as though mealtimes were part of a handrail to guide her through the day.

"I can do you cod with parsley sauce, scrambled eggs with smoked salmon or macaroni cheese," I say.

"Or we could go out for a meal," she says. She has noticed the bright spring sunshine.

I'm not offended at the apparent rejection of my lunch options. I seize the opportunity to get her dressed and out of the house before dementia stagnates her forever, slumped on the sofa in a nightdress and bathrobe.

"You'd better get dressed then," I say, and her enthusiasm wilts. The prospect of climbing upstairs is like scaling Everest.

"Suppose we draw the curtains and I get you some clothes," I say.

"Oh, that's an idea," she says, so I fetch her a bra, top, shoes and trousers. She inspects them with dementia-driven disapproval. "I'm not a hundred," she says, even though she has worn the outfit before and looked an amazing eighty-seven.

At last, she is dressed, and we take a tram into the city. Our favourite bistro is full, so I steer the wheelchair up a side alley into a square that is mostly pizza restaurants, almost empty. We are welcomed to a sunny window table where we share a tasty pizza with salad, followed by a delicious cheesecake. One cheesecake, two spoons. I smile at my wife, and she smiles back.

"What are you smiling about?" she asks.

"Just thinking how lovely this is," I say. "You and me together, in the sunshine, sharing a nice lunch. It was a good idea."

"Yes," my wife says. "It's good. Pity my husband couldn't join us."

But she's happy. Whoever she thinks I am, why should I mind?

27

Sorry, Sorry, Sorry

"Sorry," my wife says.

"Don't keep saying sorry," I say to her. I am standing behind her halfway up the stairs on our way to bed.

"I'm so slow," she says.

"You're eighty-seven," I remind her. "You're allowed to be slow."

"I'm sorry," she says again.

In the morning, I have a hospital appointment. I tell her the plan.

"What day is it?" she says.

"It's Wednesday," I say. "We're going on an adventure."

"Shall I want to go?" she asks.

"You have to come with me," I say. "I can't leave you for three or four hours on your own. I have to go to the hospital for a blood test. We take a tram to the station, get on another tram to the hospital. When I've had my blood test, we'll take a tram into the city and go out for lunch."

It's an adventure because we've never made this particular journey before, and I'm not very familiar with the trams.

"You could go on your own," she says.

"No," I say. "Besides, you need to get out, get some fresh air."

"I'm messing things up for you, aren't I? I'm sorry."

There we go again: 'Sorry'. But in a way, I'm glad because in the midst of her dementia's confusion and reluctance, there is this flash of understanding that her illness is making difficulties for me.

"I don't suppose I've got any choice," she says.

"Once you're up and dressed," I say, "and once we're on the tram, you'll enjoy it. You know you will."

It is two hours before we are ready. Waiting in the wheelchair at the tram stop, she says, "Where are we going?"

I refrain from explaining all over again the reason for the outing.

"On an adventure," I say. "Just wait and see."

She seems content with that. It is a bright, sunny day. The journey is surprisingly straightforward, and we lunch together in our favourite bistro, where the food is really good.

No arctic expedition, no tropical safari, but for us both a simple but satisfying adventure.

28
Nobody Knows – Part One

"Are you staying here tonight?" my wife asks.

"Er…yes," I say, wondering where this is going.

"Won't somebody wonder where you are?"

"Er…no. I live here. I don't have somewhere else to go."

"Do you have family?"

"Yes, you're my family. You and me, the children, my sister in Wellingborough."

"What about your parents?"

"They died," I say, "as did yours. We're orphans." But the mention of Wellingborough has kindled a flame.

"We used to live in Wellingborough," she says.

"That was a long time ago," I say.

"Can we go back there?" she asks.

"Why?" I ask her.

"Well, we can't stay here forever, can we?"

"Yes, we can. It's our home. It's where we live. It belongs to us. We can live here as long as we like."

"But what about the others?"

"Who?"

"I don't know."

We are sitting side by side on the sofa. I point the remote control at the TV and switch it off.

There is a long silence.

At last, she speaks. "What happens now?" she says.

I point to the tray of supper things on the coffee tables in front of us. "Well, if I clear these things away, I can give you your bedtime pills, and we can go to bed."

She falls silent again, and I guess from her face that she is wrestling with the possibility that 'the others' are imaginary. Then, in a moment that is totally disconnected from her dementia and in a sudden grasp of reality, she says, "The trouble is, neither of us knows what I'm talking about."

I stop to take that in, and I laugh. I stop for a moment, and then I laugh again, shaking so much I have to put the tray down.

"What are you laughing about?" she asks. And I think, *what a shame she doesn't know why it's so funny.*

29

Nobody Knows – Part Two

"Is this the one?" my wife asks.

"Yes," I say.

"Is it all right to go in?"

I have followed her upstairs, and we are on the landing, where she is tentatively putting her hand on the bedroom door handle.

"Yes," I say.

She opens the door, and there is a moment of recognition: the same pictures, the same curtains, the same bed in which we have been sleeping since we moved in nearly two years ago...

"Oh, yes," she says. "I'll use the bathroom first." So, she opens the bathroom door, and a regular bedtime ritual reasserts itself.

When I'm ready for bed, she is sitting on the edge of it, pulling on her nightdress.

"Are you sleeping here too?" she asks.

"As usual," I say.

"Oh," she says doubtfully. "Is that legal?"

"It's been legal for sixty years," I say. "Get in."

We settle down and switch off the lights. For a long time, there is silence. Then I feel a hand moving under the duvet until it finds mine and takes it.

"Are you Richard?" she asks.

"Yes," I say, and give her hand a squeeze.

"That's a relief," she says.

Silence for a while. Then I laugh.

"What's funny?" my wife says.

"I'm just remembering what you said downstairs. Neither of us know what you're talking about. You are a one."

"Am I?"

"Yes, you are, and just as well. Two of you would be unbearable."

"Oh *you*!" she says.

She releases my hand and slides a finger into the waistband of my boxer shorts, pulling it back and letting it go. It pings against my skin.

Suddenly, we have returned to 2019 B.D. – that's Before Dementia. God's in his heaven; all's right with the world. Possibly.

So, catch it while you can.

30
Trees in the Corners

"Those…erm…what do you call them?" my wife says.

"If you don't know, then I can't tell you," I reply.

"Green things," she says, exasperated. "That one, and that one," she says, hands flapping in opposite directions. "In the corners."

"Do you mean the trees?"

"Yes," she says. "How can I not know *trees*?"

"Because you've got dementia," I say. "It's a malfunction of the brain. You forget things."

"I didn't know that," she says.

"That's because you've forgotten it."

She points at the two ornamental trees in opposite corners of the room. "Those…what are they?"

"Trees," I say.

"Have they been watered?"

This is a question she asks from time to time. Suddenly, out of the blue, she asks it. It is a concern amongst others.

"Are we locked in?"

"Yes," I reply, "back and front."

Or in the kitchen, she notices a sliver of onion skin that has floated to the floor while I've been preparing a meal. She points to it with her stick. "Someone might slip on that."

I am puzzled that someone whose mind rarely focuses on anything at all and mostly spends the day not knowing what's going on unexpectedly fills the vacuum with a precisely focused question or comment.

It is an echo of when things were normal and we were about to set off on holiday and my wife would insist on tidying the house, plumping cushions, straightening rugs and putting things away in the kitchen. I would be impatiently jangling the car keys, but we didn't leave until everything in my wife's eyes was fit to return to. I have to admit that it made for a pleasant homecoming.

So, I have learned to accept and forgive my wife's pernickety and oft repeated questions.

It's normal.